BMAT Guide by Teachers

- Designed to be pedagogically effective by teachers from Singapore, the top education system in the world. Great for both weak and strong students.

- Highlights of commonly asked questions for the last decade and how to tackle them effectively and quickly. Helps students who are weak in examination skills.

- Examination-focused for maximum impact without wasting time by looking at the test specifications. Best for the last-minute crammers.

- Free additional online resources provided for owners of this book. Get continually updated resources such as essays, essay plans, practices FREE!

- Comprehensive information to make sure that all essential information is included for the latest BMAT syllabus. Never lose marks due to missing topics again!

- Proven track record with almost a decade in training workshops for the BMAT in many cities. Not written by just anyone, but by people who have been involved in the BMAT.

First Printing, 2017

ISBN-13: 978-1508496878
ISBN-10: 1508496870

39A Jalan Pemimpin
Singapore 577183
Republic of Singapore

www.bmat.sg

All enquiries are to be directed to ivan@bmat.sg

Why get this book?

This book was specially written by a teacher to help his students do well in the BMAT.

This book is dedicated to the many students who have done well in the BMAT under my tutelage over the years. Many of you have moved on to do great things in your medical studies and I'm sure you be will become great physicians in the future.

But forever remember this,

Primum non nocere.

About the author

This BMAT book is designed by Mr Ivan Gn, an experienced teacher in the top performing education system of Singapore, as part of the course to prepare students for the BMAT.

Ivan has been coaching students individually for the BMAT since 2009 who graduated from Imperial College London with a first-class honours degree and formerly taught for many years. He worked as a teacher in Singapore, one of the most successful education systems in the world.

He has conducted classes for the BMAT for several years in different cities such as Singapore, Bangkok, Jakarta, Shanghai and Hong Kong, and has completed a version of the test itself as part of his work. Students who have attended his classes have performed above the BMAT international average and many of them were offered interviews for NTU-Imperial LKCMedicine, Imperial College London as well as Cambridge and Oxford.

Visit our BMAT website at **www.bmat.sg** for extra free resources, more details and practice options.

WHY IS THE BMAT IMPORTANT?

SECTION 2: SCIENTIFIC KNOWLEDGE AND APPLICATIONS   34

SECTION 3: WRITING TASK

Introduction to the BMAT

Why is the BMAT important?

The BMAT is used for admissions into the top United Kingdom universities for various courses, including medicine, veterinary and biomedical courses. It is also used by the Singapore's Nanyang Technological University-Imperial College Lee Kong Chian School of Medicine (LKCMedicine) as well as several top medical universities in Thailand for admission.

The BMAT constitutes a <u>significant component</u> of the composite score for many universities, in additional to the primary qualifications such as the 'A'-Level or IB diploma. It is well-understood by insiders that the BMAT scores are as important as the primary qualifications in terms of the weight, but differs from university to university. A significantly good BMAT score will give you a very important advantage over other candidates when applying for courses in each of the universities around the world.

Why do you need to prepare for the BMAT?

Many students underestimate the difficulty of the BMAT, thinking that Section 1 is just "another IQ test", Section 2 will be a walk in the park because "they have learnt it in school" and Section 3 is just "another essay to write". However, this is not true.

Just like every examination, the BMAT has very clear specifications and requirements from each section. There are tricks that they commonly use in Section 1 that will cause the average student to trip. Spending time to prepare and familiarize yourself with these common pitfalls will help you score well. While Section 2 covers content already covered in your school, many of these questions in the BMAT are inter-disciplinary, the ones you will never see in school tests. Knowing how to spot these questions will put you head of the pack. Section 3 is not just another essay to write, but one with very clear requirements. You need to answer the essay question in a specific manner to cover all the requirements that will get your grade up. It is not totally an English language examination, but one of content and arguments which you can prepare for.

Do not treat the BMAT lightly, because as a test-taker you will have to finish these questions in a very short amount of time. We'll get into that later and how to manage your time properly.

BMAT Expectations

The BMAT is an extremely competitive and intensive test which covers a broad spectrum of not just content knowledge, but logical thinking and skills as well. Students are expected to be able to handle questions involving simple logic and arguments, as well as answer content questions across all three science domains of Chemistry, Biology and Physics, as well as Mathematics.

The specific requirements of the BMAT are listed below:

Knowledge

- Familiarity with concepts, terms and propositional knowledge specified by the national curriculum up to and including 'A'-Level Science (Chemistry, Biology and Physics) and Mathematics.

Skills

Handling of number and communication, specifically:

- ability to read formal English and follow written instructions;
- ability to work quickly and accurately;
- ability to perform very simple mental arithmetic;
- ability to identify the straightforward meaning of particular phrases within a longer text;
- ability to extract the meaning intended by an author where to do so requires more than one syntactical element of the text to be understood and synthesized;
- ability to read simple quantitative data presented numerically or graphically and to understand their straightforward meaning and to be able to produce simple and appropriate graphs or diagrams of quantitative data;
- ability to generalize from quantitative data, for example to interpret a trend, a pattern, or a rate and to be able to apply the generalisation to the particular or hypothetical context;
- ability to make logical inferences or deductions from textual information and quantitative data and to identify illogical inferences;
- ability to communicate knowledge, understanding, interpretation, inferences, arguments, deductions and predictions by the appropriate use of clear and concise written English and diagrams;

- tendency to take approaches that are critical, evidence-based, and which consider alternatives.

Structure of the BMAT

The test has three elements, a 60-minute test of Aptitude and Skills, a 30-minute test of Scientific Knowledge and Applications and a 30-minute Writing Task. The structure of each of these three elements is outlined below.

Test format

There will be separate question papers for each of Sections 1, 2 and 3.

Except for the Writing Task (Section 3), all questions will be in objective or semi-objective formats. Questions or sub-questions will each carry one mark, so that although clusters of sub-questions relating to the same stimulus will be feasible, partial credit items will not be used. For Sections 1 and 2, exhaustive answer keys will be finalised after inspection of the range of responses to each question; followed by automated marking, psychometric analysis, test calibration and the issue of results.

Section 1: Aptitude and Skills

This element tests generic skills often utilised in undergraduate study. The range of these and the approximate balance between them in terms of the time and number of marks which will be available is outlined below. Questions will be in multiple-choice or short answer form. Calculators may not be used.

	Minutes	Marks
Problem Solving demands insight to determine how to encode and process numerical information so as to solve problems, using simple numerical and algebraic operations. Problem solving will require the capacity to ... • select relevant information • recognise analogous cases • determine and apply appropriate procedures	30 (suggested)	13
Understanding Argument presents a series of logical arguments and requires respondents to ... • identify reasons, assumptions, & conclusions • detect flaws • draw conclusions	15 (suggested)	10

Data Analysis & Inference demands the use of information skills (vocabulary, comprehension, basic descriptive statistics and graphical tools), data interpretation, analysis and scientific inference and deduction to reach appropriate conclusions from information provided in different forms, namely ... • verbal • statistical • graphical	15 (suggested)	12
TOTAL	60	35

Section 2: Scientific Knowledge and Applications

This element tests whether candidates have the core knowledge and the capacity to apply it which is a pre-requisite for high level study in biomedical sciences. Questions will be restricted to material normally included in non-specialist school science and mathematics courses, as exemplified by the UK national curriculum for Science and Additional Science and Mathematics up to and including Key Stage 4 ('A'-Level equivalent). They will however require a level of understanding appropriate for such an able target group. The balance between the subject areas in terms of time and marks available is outlined below. Questions will be in multiple-choice or short answer form. Calculators may not be used.

	Minutes	Marks available
Biology	8 (suggested)	6-8
Physics	8 (suggested)	6-8
Chemistry	8 (suggested)	6-8
Mathematics	6 (suggested)	5-7
TOTAL	30	27

Section 3: Writing Task

A selection of four tasks will be available, from which one must be chosen. These will include brief questions based on topics of general, medical, veterinary or scientific interest.

Questions will provide a short proposition and may require candidates to:

- explain or discuss the proposition's implications;
- suggest a counter proposition or argument;
- suggest a (method for) resolution.

The Writing Task provides an opportunity for candidates to demonstrate the capacity to consider different aspects of a proposition, and to communicate them effectively in writing. Skills to be assessed include those concerning communication, described above. All specified skills may be assessed. The question paper will brief candidates about the nature and purpose of the Task. They will be required to produce a written communication, without the assistance of a dictionary or automated spelling and grammar checking software. Whilst they may make preliminary notes, the final product is strictly limited to one A4 page, to promote the disciplined selection and organisation of ideas, together with their concise, accurate and effective expression. When scoring responses, consideration will be given to the degree to which candidates have: addressed the question in the way demanded; organised their thoughts clearly; expressed themselves using concise, compelling and correct English; used their general knowledge and opinions appropriately. Admitting institutions will be provided with a copy of the applicant's response.

	Minutes
TOTAL	30

How is the BMAT scored?

Section 1 and 2

Results for Sections 1 and 2 are reported on the BMAT scale, which runs from 1 (low) to 9 (high), with scores being reported to one decimal place. Extreme scores are expected to be comparatively rare. The scale has been designed so that typical applicants to the most highly selective undergraduate university courses in the UK (who are by definition academically very able) will score around 5.0. The best applicants will score more highly, but 6.0 represents a comparatively high score and only a few very exceptional applicants will achieve BMAT scores higher than 7.0.

Section 3

Essay marks are awarded separately for the quality of content and quality of English.

BMAT Essay Marking Criteria – quality of content

In arriving at the score for quality of content, markers are instructed to consider:

- Has the candidate addressed the question in the way demanded?
- Have they organised their thoughts clearly?
- Have they used their general knowledge and opinions appropriately?

Scores are awarded on a scale from 1 to 5.

Score 1

An answer that has some bearing on the question but which does not address the question in the way demanded, is incoherent or unfocussed.

Score 2

An answer that addresses most of the components of the question and is arranged in a reasonably logical way. There may be significant elements of confusion in the argument. The candidate may misconstrue certain important aspects of the main proposition or its implication or may provide an unconvincing or weak counter proposition.

Score 3

A reasonably well-argued answer that addresses ALL aspects of the question, making reasonable use of the material provided and generating a reasonable counter-proposition or argument. The argument is relatively rational. There may be some weakness in the force of the argument or the coherence of the ideas, or some aspect of the argument may have been overlooked.

Score 4

A good answer with few weaknesses. ALL aspects of the question are addressed, making good use of the material and generating a good counter proposition or argument. The argument is rational. Ideas are expressed and arranged in a coherent way, with a balanced consideration of the proposition and counter proposition.

Score 5

An excellent answer with no significant weaknesses. ALL aspects of the question are addressed, making excellent use of the material and generating an excellent counter proposition or argument. The argument is cogent. Ideas are expressed in a clear and logical way, considering a breadth of relevant points and leading to a compelling synthesis or conclusion.

An answer judged to be irrelevant, trivial, unintelligible or missing will be given a score of 0.

BMAT Essay Marking Criteria - quality of English

In arriving at the score for quality of English, markers are instructed to consider:

Have they expressed themselves clearly using concise, compelling and correct English?

Scores are awarded on a scale from A to E.

Band A – Good use of English.

- fluent
- good sentence structure
- good use of vocabulary
- sound use of grammar
- good spelling and punctuation
- few slips or errors

Band C – Reasonably clear use of English.

- There may be some weakness in the effectiveness of the English.
- reasonably fluent/not difficult to read
- simple/unambiguous sentence structure
- fair range and appropriate use of vocabulary
- acceptable grammar
- reasonable spelling and punctuation
- some slips/errors

Band E – Rather weak use of English.

- hesitant fluency/not easy to follow at times
- some flawed sentence structure/paragraphing
- limited range of vocabulary
- faulty grammar
- regular spelling/punctuation errors
- regular and frequent slips or errors

An essay that is judged to be below the level of an E will receive an X.

Each essay is double marked. For each scale, if the two scores awarded are the same or occupy adjacent positions on the scale, the scores are combined to give the final mark. If there is a larger discrepancy in the scores on either of the two scales, the essay is marked for a third time, and the final mark awarded is checked by the BMAT Assessment Manager.

The composite mark for the quality of English is derived by combining the two scores as follows: AA = A, AC = B, CC = C, CE = D, EE = E. The composite mark for the quality of content is derived by calculating the average of the two scores.

Visit **http://www.bmat.sg** to download free essays!

Section 1: Aptitude and Skills

The three main skills tested in this section are:

1. Problem solving;
2. Understanding argument;
3. Data analysis and inference.

The level of mathematics required in this section is up to GCSE or 'O'-Levels, so most of the skills required will not be technical in nature. In fact, it is more like an IQ test which will test your ability to think clearly, break complex problems down into smaller problems and recognise patterns.

Tackling Problem Solving Questions

These questions test you on your ability to understand, compare, use and analyse mathematical information. Sometimes numerical data is given, sometimes graphs and other visual representations of data is provided.

You are expected to be able to identify the sets of data which are relevant and important to solving the given question. Expect to be given other data which are not important to distract and confuse you.

You will also be expected to be able to recognise patterns and cases which are similar to each other that can be applied similarly. This includes the ability to recognise cause and effect in data and identify reasons for possible trends in data.

There is no easy way to teach you how to solve these problem-solving questions. You will notice some trends after practicing the past year papers that certain types of questions regularly repeat.

Tackling Argument Questions

The Structure of Arguments

In order to understand the strengths and weaknesses of arguments, it is important for you to learn the basic of logic and the structure of arguments.

The proposition is the basic unit of what may be asserted or denied that is typically written as a declarative sentence.

Propositions are different from the sentences that convey them. "Alvin loves Jane" expresses exactly the same proposition as "Jane is loved by Alvin," while the sentence "Today is my birthday" can be used to convey many different propositions, depending upon who happens to utter it, and on what day. But each proposition is either true or false. Sometimes, we don't know whether a proposition is true or false, but we can be sure that it has one or the other.

The main issue of logic is how the truth of some propositions is related to the truth of another. As such, we will usually consider a group of related propositions called arguments. An <u>argument</u> is a set of two or more propositions related to each other in such a way that all but one of them, we call the <u>premises</u>, are supposed to provide support for the remaining one, which we call the <u>conclusion</u>. The transition from premises to conclusion, the logical connection between them, is the inference upon which the argument relies. In order to understand the logic of argument, you must understand the ideas behind the premises and the conclusion above.

Notice that "premise" and "conclusion" are here defined only as they occur in relation to each other within a particular argument. One and the same proposition can (and often does) appear as the conclusion of one line of reasoning but also as one of the premises of another. Different words and phrases are used to indicate the premises and conclusion of an argument, although their use is never strictly required, since the context can make clear the direction of movement.

Therefore the following, "The beach is full of sand, and I love apples. My dog loves to chase cats." is just a collection of unrelated propositions; the truth or falsity of each has no bearing on that of the others.

But "Daniel is a doctor, so Daniel must have gone to medical school since all doctors have to be trained in medical schools" is an argument; the truth of its conclusion, " Daniel must have gone to medical school," is inferentially derived from its premises, "Daniel is a doctor." and " all doctors have to be trained in medical school."

Recognizing Arguments

As many BMAT questions deal with arguments, it's important to identify the arguments in the BMAT texts and to identify which proposition is the conclusion of each argument, since that's a necessary step in the analysis of the inference that is supposed to lead to it. It is possible employ a simple diagram to represent the structure of an argument, numbering each of the propositions it comprises and drawing an arrow to indicate the inference that leads from its premise(s) to its conclusion.

You should be able to tell the difference between an argument and a mere collection of propositions and to identify the intended conclusion of each argument.

Remember the basic definition of an argument: it includes more than one proposition, and it infers a conclusion from one or more premises. So "If John has already left, then either Jane has arrived or Tom is on the way." can't be an argument, since it is just one big (compound) proposition. But "John has already left, since Jane has arrived." is an argument that proposes an inference from the fact of Jane's arrival to the conclusion, "John has already left." If you find it helpful to draw a diagram, please make good use of that method to your advantage in the BMAT. You will learn some examples of how we use such diagrams to illustrate the logic of the argument questions.

Our primary concern is to evaluate the reliability of inferences, the patterns of reasoning that lead from premises to conclusion in a logical argument. It is vital from the outset to distinguish two kinds of inference, each of which has its own distinctive structure and standard of correctness.

Deductive Inferences

When an argument claims that the truth of its premises guarantees the truth of its conclusion, it is said to involve a deductive inference. Deductive reasoning holds to a very high standard of correctness. A deductive inference succeeds only if its premises provide such absolute and complete support for its conclusion that it would be utterly inconsistent to suppose that the premises are true but the conclusion false.

Notice that each argument either meets this standard or else it does not; there is no middle ground. Some deductive arguments are perfect, and if their premises are in fact true, then it follows that their conclusions must also be true, no matter what else may happen to be the case. All other deductive arguments are no good at all—their conclusions may be false even if their premises are true, and no amount of additional information can help them in the least.

Inductive Inferences

When an argument claims merely that the truth of its premises make it likely or probable that its conclusion is also true, it is said to involve an inductive inference. The standard of correctness for inductive reasoning is much more flexible than that for deduction. An inductive argument succeeds whenever its premises provide some legitimate evidence or support for the truth of its conclusion. Although it is therefore reasonable to accept the truth of that conclusion on these grounds, it would not be completely inconsistent to withhold judgment or even to deny it outright.

Inductive arguments, then, may meet their standard to a greater or to a lesser degree, depending upon the amount of support they supply. No inductive argument is either absolutely perfect or entirely useless, although one may be said to be relatively better or worse than another in the sense that it recommends its conclusion with a higher or lower degree of probability. In such cases, relevant additional information often affects the reliability of an inductive argument by providing other evidence that changes our estimation of the likelihood of the conclusion.

It should be possible to differentiate arguments of these two sorts with some accuracy already. Remember that deductive arguments claim to guarantee their conclusions, while inductive arguments merely recommend theirs. Or ask yourself whether the introduction of any additional information—short of changing or denying any of the premises—could make the conclusion seem more or less likely; if so, the pattern of reasoning is inductive.

Truth and Validity

Since deductive reasoning requires such a strong relationship between premises and conclusion, we will spend most section studying various patterns of deductive inference. It is therefore worthwhile to consider the standard of correctness for deductive arguments in some detail.

A deductive argument is said to be valid when the inference from premises to conclusion is perfect. Here are two equivalent ways of stating that standard:

If the premises of a valid argument are true, then its conclusion must also be true.

It is impossible for the conclusion of a valid argument to be false while its premises are true.

(Considering the premises as a set of propositions, we will say that the premises are true only on those occasions when each and every one of those propositions is true.)

Any deductive argument that is not valid is invalid: it is possible for its conclusion to be false while its premises are true, so even if the premises are true, the conclusion may turn out to be either true or false.

Premises	Inference	Conclusion
True	Valid	True
		XXXX
	Invalid	True
		False
False	Valid	True
		False
	Invalid	True
		False

The validity of the inference of a deductive argument is independent of the truth of its premises; both conditions must be met in order to be sure of the truth of the conclusion. Of the eight distinct possible combinations of truth and validity, only one is ruled out completely:

The only thing that cannot happen is for a deductive argument to have true premises and a valid inference but a false conclusion.

Some logicians designate the combination of true premises and a valid inference as a sound argument; it is a piece of reasoning whose conclusion must be true. The trouble with every other case is that it gets us nowhere, since either at least one of the premises is false, or the inference is invalid, or both. The conclusions of such arguments may be either true or false, so they are entirely useless in any effort to gain additional information.

Common Fallacies

Listed here are some common logical fallacies which affect the validity of arguments. For the BMAT, you are not required to know the names of the fallacies. It is useful to be to recognise the flaws in the fallacious arguments presented in the scenarios given in the questions. These are the most common fallacies that appear in the BMAT, and if you can recognize them quickly you will be able to use them better in the BMAT.

Hasty generalization

Definition: Making assumptions about a whole group or range of cases based on a sample that is atypical or too small. Stereotypes about people ("scientists are shy and smart," "wealthy people are snobs," etc.) are a common example of the principle underlying hasty generalization.

Example: "My roommate says that fast food is tasty, and this fast food that I'm having is tasty too. Therefore all fast food must be tasty!" Two people's experiences are, in this case, not enough on which to base a conclusion.

How to recognize this in the BMAT: Statement uses a single or a few examples to draw a conclusion that covered everything.

Missing the point

Definition: The premises of an argument do support a particular conclusion—but not the conclusion that the arguer actually draws.

Example: "The seriousness of a punishment should match the seriousness of the crime. Right now, the punishment for drunk driving may simply be a fine. But drunk driving is a very serious crime that can kill innocent people. So the death penalty should be the punishment for drunk driving." The argument actually supports several conclusions—"The punishment for drunk driving should be very serious," in particular—but it doesn't support the claim that the death penalty, specifically, is warranted.

False cause

Definition: Assuming that because B comes after A, A caused B. Of course, sometimes one event really does cause another one that comes later—for example, if I register for a class, and my name later appears on the roll, it's true that the first event caused the one that came later. But sometimes two events that seem related in time aren't really related as cause and event. That is, correlation isn't the same thing as causation.

Examples: "President Jones raised taxes, and then the rate of violent crime went up. Jones is responsible for the rise in crime." The increase in taxes might or might not be one factor in the rising crime rates, but the argument hasn't shown us that one caused the other.

How to recognize this in the BMAT: A statement that shows no proof of cause and effect, simply stating it due to the order of events.

Slippery slope

Definition: The arguer claims that a sort of chain reaction, usually ending in some dire consequence, will take place, but there's really not enough evidence for that assumption. The arguer asserts that if we take even one step onto the "slippery slope," we will end up sliding all the way to the bottom; he or she assumes we can't stop partway down the hill.

Example: "Animal experimentation reduces our respect for life. If we don't respect life, we are likely to be more and more tolerant of violent acts like war and murder. Soon our society will become a battlefield in which everyone constantly fears for their lives. It will be the end of civilization. To prevent this terrible consequence, we should make animal experimentation illegal right now." Since animal experimentation has been legal for some time and civilization has not yet ended, it seems particularly clear that this chain of events won't necessarily take place. Even if we believe that experimenting on animals reduces respect for life, and loss of respect for life makes us more tolerant of violence, that may be the spot on the hillside at which things stop—we may not slide all the way down to the end of civilization. And so we have not yet been given sufficient reason to accept the arguer's conclusion that we must make animal experimentation illegal right now.

Like post hoc, slippery slope can be a tricky fallacy to identify, since sometimes a chain of events really can be predicted to follow from a certain action. Here's an example that doesn't seem fallacious: "If I fail English 101, I won't be able to graduate. If I don't graduate, I probably won't be able to get a good job, and I may very well end up doing temp work or flipping burgers for the next year."

How to recognize this in the BMAT: A series of hypothetical consequences given from a single event, all of which have concrete proof of actually happening.

Weak analogy

Definition: Many arguments rely on an analogy between two or more objects, ideas, or situations. If the two things that are being compared aren't really alike in the relevant respects, the analogy is a weak one, and the argument that relies on it commits the fallacy of weak analogy.

Example: "Guns are like hammers—they're both tools with metal parts that could be used to kill someone. And yet it would be ridiculous to restrict the purchase of hammers—so restrictions on purchasing guns are equally ridiculous." While guns and hammers do share certain features, these features (having metal parts, being tools, and being potentially useful for violence) are not the ones at stake in deciding whether to restrict guns. Rather, we restrict guns because they can easily be used to kill large numbers of people at a distance. This is a feature hammers do not share—it would be hard to kill a crowd with a hammer. Thus, the analogy is weak, and so is the argument based on it.

If you think about it, you can make an analogy of some kind between almost any two things in the world: "My paper is like a mud puddle because they both get bigger when it rains (I work more when I'm stuck inside) and they're both kind of murky." So the mere fact that you can draw an analogy between two things doesn't prove much, by itself.

Arguments by analogy are often used in discussing abortion—arguers frequently compare fetuses with adult human beings, and then argue that treatment that would violate the rights of an adult human being also violates the rights of fetuses. Whether these arguments are good or not depends on the strength of the analogy: do adult humans and fetuses share the properties that give adult humans rights? If the property that matters is having a human genetic code or the potential for a life full of human experiences, adult humans and fetuses do share that property, so the argument and the analogy are strong; if the property is being self-aware, rational, or able to survive on one's own, adult humans and fetuses don't share it, and the analogy is weak.

How to recognize this in the BMAT: Statements that use analogies which may not be appropriate.

Appeal to authority

Definition: Often we add strength to our arguments by referring to respected sources or authorities and explaining their positions on the issues we're discussing. If, however, we try to get readers to agree with us simply by impressing them with a famous name or by appealing to a supposed authority who really isn't much of an expert, we commit the fallacy of appeal to authority.

Example: "We should abolish the death penalty. Many respected people, such as actor Guy Handsome, have publicly stated their opposition to it." While Guy Handsome may be an authority on matters having to do with acting, there's no particular reason why anyone should be moved by his political opinions—he is probably no more of an authority on the death penalty than the person writing the paper.

How to recognize this in the BMAT: Statements use proof by referring to the opinions of respected sources such as scientists and other experts instead of referring to facts.

Ad populum

Definition: The Latin name of this fallacy means "to the people." There are several versions of the AD POPULUM fallacy, but what they all have in common is that in them, the arguer takes advantage of the desire most people have to be liked and to fit in with others and uses that desire to try to get the audience to accept his or her argument. One of the most common versions is the bandwagon fallacy, in which the arguer tries to convince the audience to do or believe something because everyone else (supposedly) does.

Example: "Gay marriages are just immoral. 70% of Americans think so!" While the opinion of most Americans might be relevant in determining what laws we should have, it certainly doesn't determine what is moral or immoral: there was a time where a substantial number of Americans were in favor of segregation, but their opinion was not evidence that segregation was moral. The arguer is trying to get us to agree with the conclusion by appealing to our desire to fit in with other Americans.

How to recognize this in the BMAT: Statements that advocate that an opinion must be right because the majority of people say so.

Ad hominem and tu quoque

Definitions: Like the appeal to authority and ad populum fallacies, the ad hominem ("against the person") and tu quoque ("you, too!") fallacies focus our attention on people rather than on arguments or evidence. In both of these arguments, the conclusion is usually "You shouldn't believe So-and-So's argument." The reason for not believing So-and-So is that So-and-So is either a bad person (ad hominem) or a hypocrite (tu quoque). in an ad hominem argument, the arguer attacks his or her opponent instead of the opponent's argument.

Examples: "Andrea Kilburn has written several books arguing that pornography harms women. But Kilburn is just ugly and bitter, so why should we listen to her?" Kilburn's appearance and character, which the arguer has characterized so ungenerously, have nothing to do with the strength of her argument, so using them as evidence is fallacious.

In a tu quoque argument, the arguer points out that the opponent has actually done the thing he or she is arguing against, and so the opponent's argument shouldn't be listened to. Here's an example: imagine that your parents have explained to you why you shouldn't smoke, and they've given a lot of good reasons—the damage to your health, the cost, and so forth. You reply, "I won't accept your argument, because you used to smoke when you were my age. You did it, too!" The fact that your parents have done the thing they are condemning has no bearing on the premises they put forward in their argument (smoking harms your health and is very expensive), so your response is fallacious.

How to recognize this in the BMAT: Statements that dispute facts by discrediting people instead of attacking the facts themselves.

Appeal to pity

Definition: The appeal to pity takes place when an arguer tries to get people to accept a conclusion by making them feel sorry for someone.

Examples: "I know the exam is graded based on performance, but you should give me an A. My cat has been sick, my car broke down, and I've had a cold, so it was really hard for me to study!" The conclusion here is "You should give me an A." But the criteria for getting an A have to do with learning and applying the material from the course; the principle the arguer wants us to accept (people who have a hard week deserve A's) is clearly unacceptable. The information the arguer has given might FEEL relevant and might even get the audience to consider the conclusion—but the information isn't logically relevant, and so the argument is fallacious. Here's another example: "It's wrong to tax corporations—think of all the money they give to charity, and of the costs they already pay to run their businesses!"

How to recognize this in the BMAT: Statements that advocate an opinion is correct because the of the sorry and pitiful state of the people affected by it.

Appeal to ignorance

Definition: In the appeal to ignorance, the arguer basically says, "Look, there's no conclusive evidence on the issue at hand. Therefore, you should accept my conclusion on this issue."

Example: "People have been trying for centuries to prove that God exists. But no one has yet been able to prove it. Therefore, God does not exist." Here's an opposing argument that commits the same fallacy: "People have been trying for years to prove that God does not exist. But no one has yet been able to prove it. Therefore, God exists." In each case, the arguer tries to use the lack of evidence as support for a positive claim about the truth of a conclusion. There is one situation in which doing this is not fallacious: if qualified researchers have used well-thought-out methods to search for something for a long time, they haven't found it, and it's the kind of thing people ought to be able to find, then the fact that they haven't found it constitutes some evidence that it doesn't exist.

Straw man

Definition: One way of making our own arguments stronger is to anticipate and respond in advance to the arguments that an opponent might make. In the straw man fallacy, the arguer sets up a weak version of the opponent's position and tries to score points by knocking it down. But just as being able to knock down a straw man (like a scarecrow) isn't very impressive, defeating a watered-down version of your opponent's argument isn't very impressive either.

Example: "Feminists want to ban all pornography and punish everyone who looks at it! But such harsh measures are surely inappropriate, so the feminists are wrong: porn and its fans should be left in peace." The feminist argument is made weak by being overstated. In fact, most feminists do not propose an outright "ban" on porn or any punishment for those who merely view it or approve of it; often, they propose some restrictions on particular things like child porn, or propose to allow people who are hurt by porn to sue publishers and producers—not viewers—for damages. So the arguer hasn't really scored any points; he or she has just committed a fallacy.

How to recognize this in the BMAT: Changing the original propositions in the statement by making it weaker and easier to attack.

Red herring

Definition: Partway through an argument, the arguer goes off on a tangent, raising a side issue that distracts the audience from what's really at stake. Often, the arguer never returns to the original issue.

Example: "Grading this exam on a curve would be the fairest thing to do. After all, classes go more smoothly when the students and the professor are getting along well." Let's try our premise-conclusion outlining to see what's wrong with this argument:

Premise: Classes go more smoothly when the students and the professor are getting along well.

Conclusion: Grading this exam on a curve would be the fairest thing to do.

When we lay it out this way, it's pretty obvious that the arguer went off on a tangent—the fact that something helps people get along doesn't necessarily make it fairer; fairness and justice sometimes require us to do things that cause conflict. But the audience may feel like the issue of teachers and students agreeing is important and be distracted from the fact that the arguer has not given any evidence as to why a curve would be fair.

How to recognize this in the BMAT: Statements with no relationships between the premises and the conclusions.

False dichotomy

Definition: In false dichotomy, the arguer sets up the situation so it looks like there are only two choices. The arguer then eliminates one of the choices, so it seems that we are left with only one option: the one the arguer wanted us to pick in the first place. But often there are really many different options, not just two—and if we thought about them all, we might not be so quick to pick the one the arguer recommends.

Example: "Caldwell Hall is in bad shape. Either we tear it down and put up a new building, or we continue to risk students' safety. Obviously we shouldn't risk anyone's safety, so we must tear the building down." The argument neglects to mention the possibility that we might repair the building or find some way to protect students from the risks in question—for example, if only a few rooms are in bad shape, perhaps we shouldn't hold classes in those rooms.

How to recognize this in the BMAT: Statements which present only a few options that the author wants you to think are the only options. However, there are other options which have intentionally be hidden from you.

Begging the question

Definition: A complicated fallacy; it comes in several forms and can be harder to detect than many of the other fallacies we've discussed. Basically, an argument that begs the question asks the reader to simply accept the conclusion without providing real evidence; the argument either relies on a premise that says the same thing as the conclusion (which you might hear referred to as "being circular" or "circular reasoning"), or simply ignores an important (but questionable) assumption that the argument rests on. Sometimes people use the phrase "beg the question" as a sort of general criticism of arguments, to mean that an arguer hasn't given very good reasons for a conclusion, but that's not the meaning we're going to discuss here.

Examples: "Active euthanasia is morally acceptable. It is a decent, ethical thing to help another human being escape suffering through death." Let's lay this out in premise-conclusion form:

Premise: It is a decent, ethical thing to help another human being escape suffering through death.

Conclusion: Active euthanasia is morally acceptable.

"Decent, ethical" means pretty much the same thing as "morally acceptable," and "help another human being escape suffering through death" means something pretty similar to "active euthanasia." So the premise basically says, "active euthanasia is morally acceptable," just like the conclusion does.

How to recognize this in the BMAT: The meaning of the premise and the conclusion is the same, only worded differently.

Section 2: Scientific Knowledge and Applications

Mathematics

Basic arithmetic

Basic arithmetic is required, as no calculators are allowed in the BMAT. You would be expected to know basic mathematical operations and the order of operations.

- The BIDMAS rule (Brackets, Indices, Division, Multiplication, Addition, and Subtraction) tells you the order to carry out mathematical operations.

Indices

- $A^0 = 1$
- $A^n \times A^m = A^{(n+m)}$
- $A^n / A^m = A^{(n-m)}$
- $A^{-n} = 1/A^n$

Surds

- $\sqrt{(A \times B)} = \sqrt{A} \times \sqrt{B}$
- $\sqrt{\left(\frac{A}{B}\right)} = \frac{\sqrt{A}}{\sqrt{B}}$

Logarithms

- If $x = b^y$, then $\log_b x = y$
- $\log_b (xy) = \log_b x + \log_b y$
- $\log_b (x/y) = \log_b x - \log_b y$

Arithmetic Series

- Series with a common difference between consecutive numbers: A, (A+ d), (A+2d)…
- N^{th} term $= A+(n-1)d$
- Sum of series up to n^{th} term $= n \times \dfrac{2A+(n-1)d}{2n}$

Geometric Series

- Series with consecutive number increasing or decreasing by a common ratio: A, Ar, Ar^2 …
- Nth term $= Ar^{(n-1)}$
- Sum of series $= A \times \dfrac{r^n - 1}{r-1}$

Significant Figures

- All non-zero digits are considered significant. For example, 92 has two significant figures (9 and 2), while 123.45 has five significant figures (1, 2, 3, 4 and 5).
- Zeros appearing anywhere between two non-zero digits are significant. Example: 101.1203 has seven significant figures: 1, 0, 1, 1, 2, 0 and 3.
- Leading zeros are not significant. For example, 0.00052 has two significant figures: 5 and 2.

Standard Form

- In standard form, a number is always written as: $A \times 10^n$
- A is always between 1 and 10. n tells us how many places to move the decimal point.

Percentage Changes

- Percentage Change = (change in value)/(original value) x 100%

Areas

- Area of square with side $A = A^2$
- Parallelogram = base x height
- Triangle = ½ x base x height
- Trapezium = ½ x (sum of parallel sides) x height
- Circle with radius $r = \pi r^2$
- Sphere = $4 \pi r^2$

Perimeters

- Square with side $A = 4A$
- Circle with radius $r = 2\pi r$

Volumes of Solids

- Cube with side $r = r^3$
- Uniform prism = area of cross-section x height
- Sphere = $4/3 \ \pi r^3$
- Cone or pyramid = $1/3$ x base area x height

Simultaneous Equations

- Substitution method. Make one equation in terms of X, substitute into the other equation to solve for Y.
- Elimination method. Multiply each equation until a common value of X is obtained. Subtract one equation from another.

Quadratic Equations

- For an equation $ax^2 + bx + c = 0$
- $$x = \frac{-b \pm \sqrt{b^2 - 4ac}}{2a}$$

Angles and Lines

- Where two lines intersect, the opposite angles are equal.
- Angles on a straight line add up to 180 degrees.
- Angles around a point add up to 360 degrees.

Triangle Rules

- Angles in a triangle add up to 180 degrees.
- A scalene triangle has three sides of different lengths
- An equilateral triangle has three sides of the same length, and internal angles are all 60 degrees.
- An isosceles triangle has two sides of the same length, and two equal angles.
- Right angle triangle has one angle of 90 degrees.

Polygon Rules

- Sum of interior angles for polygon with n sides = 180 (n-2) degrees.
- Interior angles for polygon with n sides of equal length = 180 (n-2)/n degrees.

Pythagoras Theoreom

- For a triangle with the longest side length c (hypotenuse), and two other sides of a and b.
- $a^2 + b^2 = c^2$

Trigonometry Functions

- Only valid for right-angled triangles.
- sin θ = opposite / hypotenuse
- cos θ = adjacent / hypotenuse
- tan θ = opposite / adjacent

Sine Law

- $$\frac{a}{sinA} = \frac{b}{sinB} = \frac{c}{sinC}$$

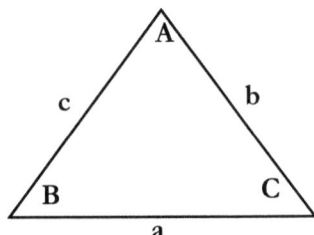

Cosine Law

- $a^2 = b^2 + c^2 - 2bc\ cosA$

Circle Theorems

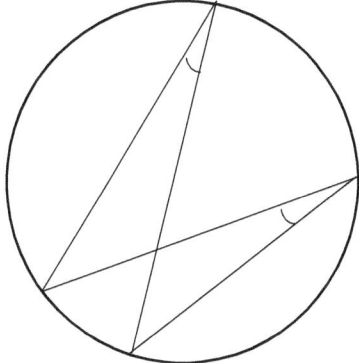

Angles formed from two points on the circumference are equal to other angles, in the same arc, formed from those two points.

- Angle in a Semi-Circle

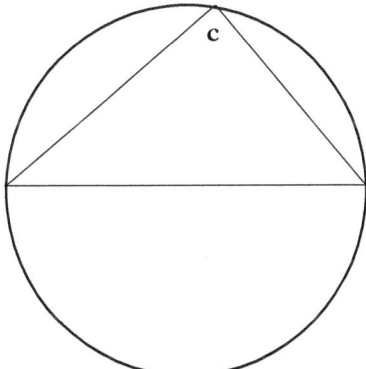

Angles formed by drawing lines from the ends of the diameter of a circle to its circumference form a right angle. So angle c is a right angle.

- Angle at the Centre

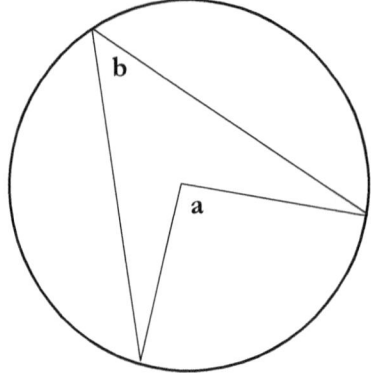

The angle formed at the centre of the circle by lines originating from two points on the circle's circumference is double the angle formed on the circumference of the circle by lines originating from the same points. i.e. a = 2b.

- Alternate Segment Theorem

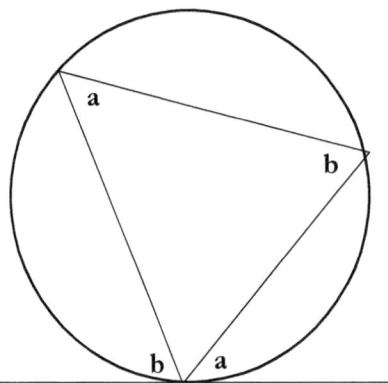

Tangent to the circle

This diagram shows the alternate segment theorem. In short, the "a" angles are equal to each other and the "b" angles are equal to each other.

Physics

SI units

- The ampere (A) - unit of measurement of electric current
- The kilogram (kg) - unit of measurement of mass
- The metre (m) - unit of measurement of length
- The second (s) - unit of measurement of time
- The kelvin (K) - unit of measurement of thermodynamic temperature
- The mole (mol) - unit of measurement of amount of substance
- The candela (cd) - unit of measurement of luminous intensity

SI prefixes

Text	Symbol	Factor
tera	T	1000000000000
giga	G	1000000000
mega	M	1000000
kilo	k	1000
hecto	h	100
deca	da	10
(none)	(none)	1
deci	d	0.1
centi	c	0.01
milli	m	0.001
micro	μ	0.000001
nano	n	0.000000001
pico	p	0.000000000001

Equations of Motion

- The equations of motion relate to the following five quantities:
    - u - initial velocity (units: m s^{-1})
    - v - final velocity (units: m s^{-1})
    - a – acceleration (units: m s^{-2})
    - t – time (units: s)
    - s – displacement (units: m)
    - Of the above u, v, a, and s are vector quantities. As such, remember to make vectors going in one direction positive and vectors in the opposite direction negative.
    - Time (t) is a scalar quantity.
    - If any three of the five quantities are known then the other two may be calculated using the following three equations:
    - $v = u + at$
    - $s = ut + \frac{1}{2}at^2$
    - $v^2 = u^2 + 2as$
- Average speed = distance travelled / time taken
- Average velocity = displacement (s) / time taken (t)
- Acceleration (a) = change in velocity (v-u)/ time taken(t)

Projectile Motion

- In projectile motion, the horizontal motion and the vertical motion are independent of each other; that is, neither motion affects the other.
- Substitute g (acceleration due to gravity) for a, and h (height) for s in the three equations above.
    - $v = u + gt$
    - $h = ut + \frac{1}{2}gt^2$
    - $v^2 = u^2 + 2gh$

Newton's Law of Force and Motion

- First Law: a body remains stationary or in uniform motion unless acted on by a force.

- Second Law: Force (units: N) = mass (units: kg) x acceleration (units: m s^{-2})
- Acceleration due to gravity is approximately 9.81 m s^{-2}
- Third Law: Action force and reaction are equal and opposite.

Force, work, power and energy

- Work done (w, units: J) = force (F, units: N) x distance <u>moved in direction</u> of the force (d, units: m) = Fd
- Power is rate of work done (units: J s^{-1}) = work done / time taken = w/t
- Energy is the capacity to do work (units: J).
- Kinetic energy (KE) is the energy of motion (units: J) = ½ x mass x velocity x velocity = ½mv^2
- Potential energy (PE) is stored energy and can exist in different forms such as gravitational potential energy (GPE), chemical potential energy (CPE) and elastic potential energy (EPE).
- For a gravitation potential energy (GPE), E = mass (units: kg) x acceleration due to gravity (units: m s^{-2}) x height (units: m) = mgh.

Force, Momentum and Impulse

- Momentum = mass x velocity = mv
- In an elastic collision, momentum and energy is conserved. The total amount of momentum before and after the collisions between the objects is the same.

$$m_1 u_1 + m_2 u_2 = m_1 v_1 + m_2 v_2$$

$$\frac{1}{2}(m_1 u_1^2 + m_2 u_2^2) = \frac{1}{2}(m_1 v_1^2 + m_2 v_2^2)$$

- In an inelastic collision, momentum is conserved, but there is some energy loss.

Force, Stress and Strain

- Stress = force / area
- Strain = extension / length
- Young's modulus of material = stress / strain
- Hooke's Law:
    - Force = -kx
    - k is the spring constant (units: $N\ m^{-1}$)
    - x is the extension of the spring (units: m)
    - Work done = $\frac{1}{2}\ kx^2$

Moments and Machines

- Moment of a force about a pivot = force x perpendicular distance from the pivot.
- For a balanced lever, the sum of the clockwise moments = anti-clockwise moments.
- Efficiency = work output / energy input

Pressure, Buoyancy and Flow

- Solids: pressure = Force / Area
- Fluids: pressure = force / area = mg / A, where m = density of the fluid x volume of fluid.
- Archimedes' Principle: Archimedes' principle indicates that the upward buoyant force that is exerted on a body immersed in a fluid, whether fully or partially submerged, is equal to the weight of the fluid that the body displaces.
- Upthrust = density of fluid x volume of fluid displaced x acceleration due to gravity
- Flow rate = volume of fluid through a cross-section / time

Gas Laws

- Boyle's Law: pressure x volume = constant.
- Charles' Law: volume / temperature = constant.
- Pressure Law: pressure / temperature = constant.
- Combined gas law: $\frac{pV}{T} = constant$
- Temperature is measured in K.
- Avogrado's Law: pV = nRT (R is the universal gas constant, n is the number of moles of gas.)
- Dalton's Law of Partial Pressure: Total pressure in a mixture of gases is the sum of the pressure of each gas.
- Henry's Law: The solubility of a gas in contact with a liquid is proportional to the partial pressure.
- Graham's Law: The rate of diffusion of a gas is inversely proportional to the square root of its molecular mass.
- Fick's First Law: The rate of diffusion of a gas is proportional to the surface area and the concentration gradient and inversely proportional to the distance.

Heat and Energy

- The specific heat capacity (c) of a substance is the amount of energy needed to change the temperature of 1 kg of the substance by 1°C. Different substances have different specific heat capacities.
- Energy required to raise m grams of a substance by ΔT, $Q = mc\Delta T$
- Specific latent heat of vapourisation is the enthalpy change required to transform one gram of a substance from a liquid into a gas at a given pressure without a change in temperature.
- Specific latent heat of fusion is the enthalpy change required to transform one gram of a substance from a solid into a liquid at a given pressure without a change in temperature.
- Heat transfers by convection, conduction and radiation.

Waves

- Two types of waves: transverse (light and electromagnetic waves) or longitudinal (sound).
- Parts of the electromagnetic (EM) wave spectrum are radio waves, microwaves, IR, visible light, UV, X-rays, gamma.
- Typical wavelengths of different parts of the EM waves:
    - Radio waves = 10^3 m
    - Microwave = 10^{-2} m
    - Infrared = 10^{-5} m`
    - Visible = 10^{-6} m
    - UV = 10^{-8} m
    - X-Ray = 10^{-10} m
    - Gamma = 10^{-12} m

- Velocity of a wave (v, units: m s^{-1}) = frequency (f) x wave length (λ) = $f\lambda$
- In reflection of a wave in the same medium, angle of incidence = angle of reflection.
- Refraction of a wave occurs when waves move from one medium to another. This results in the slowing of a wave, resulting in the bending of waves. For i = angle of incidence, and r = angle of refraction, and n = refractive index: $n = (\sin i)/(\sin r)$
- For total internal refraction to occur, the angle of the incidence > critical angle.

Electricity

- Any two charged objects will create a force on each other. Opposite charges will produce an attractive force while similar charges will produce a repulsive force.
- Coulomb's Law:
    - $F = \frac{kQ_1Q_2}{r^2}$
    - Potential difference, $1V = 1J\ C^{-1}$
- Charges can be stored between two charged plates separated by insulating material, known as capacitors.

- Capacitance (C)= charge stored / volt = Q/V
- Energy stored in capacitor = ½ CV^2
- Current, I = charge / time
- Power, P = current x voltage
- Energy = power x time
- Ohm's Law:
    - Voltage, V = current x resistance
    - Power loss, W = $current^2$ x resistance
- Effective resistance for resistors in series, R = R1 + R2 + R3...
- Effective resistance for resistors in parallel, R : 1/R = 1/R1 + 1/R2 + 1/R3...
- Effective voltage for batteries in series, E = E1 + E2 + ...
- Transformers can change the voltage and current of electricity being transmitted. The primary (V_p, before transformation) and secondary voltages (V_s, after transformation) can be calculated using the following formula: $\frac{V_p}{V_s} = \frac{n_p}{n_s}$

Radioactive Decay

- There is always background radiation reading even without a radioactive source present.
- Alpha decay, or α-decay, is a type of radioactive decay in which an atomic nucleus emits an alpha particle and thereby transforms (or 'decays') into an atom with a mass number 4 less and atomic number 2 less. It is highly polarising and weakly penetrating, typically unable to penetrate through even a piece of paper or a short distance in air. An example is given below:

$$^{238}_{92}U \rightarrow ^{234}_{90}Th + ^{4}_{2}He$$

- Beta decay releases high energy electrons. Beta radiation is more penetrating and can be blocked by a thin sheet of metal. An example is given below:

$$^{14}_{6}C \rightarrow ^{14}_{7}N + e^{-}$$

- Gamma decay is highly penetrating and weakly polarising. <u>A thick piece of lead or other dense metals</u> is typically used to stop the radiation.
- Half-time is the time taken for a radioactive material to decay to half its original amount.

Chemistry

Atomic Structure

- Atoms are consist of a nucleus of protons and neutrons, with electrons existing in orbitals around the nucleus.
- The mass number of an atom is the sum of the protons and neutrons in the nucleus.
- The proton number is the number of protons in the nucleus.
- A neutral atom has the same number of protons and electrons.
- An ion is formed if the number of protons and electrons is different.
- Electronic configuration of an atom is the arrangement of the electrons in different orbitals (s, p, d, f) and shells (n).
- S-orbitals can only contain 2 electrons, p-orbitals can contain 6, d-orbitals can have 10, while f-orbitals can have 14.

Periodicity

- Columns in the periodic table are known as groups. All the elements in the same group tend to react in a similar manner due to the fact that they have the same number of electrons in the outermost shell.
- Rows in the periodic table are known as periods. Across a period, there is usually a gradual trend of changing chemical and/or physical properties due to the change in the number of outermost electrons or the mass of the atoms.
- Group 1 is known as the alkali metals, which are extremely reactive. They will react with water vigorously to form strong alkali solutions. These metals will also tend to form ions of +1 charge. The metals are soft and tarnish in air(oxygen) quickly.
- Group 2 is known as the alkali earth metals, which are slightly less reactive than group 1 metals. They will react with water vigorously to form strong alkali solutions. These metals will also tend to form ions of +2 charge.
- Together, group 1 and 2 is known as the s-block.

- Elements in group 3 to 12 are known as the transition metals, and they are collectively known as the d-block, due to the presence of electrons in their d-orbitals. They typically have high melting points, high strength, are good electrical and heat conductors and give coloured solutions when dissolved in water. They also often exhibit variable oxidation states.
- Elements in group 13 to 17 are collectively known as p-block elements, and are typically metalloids and non-metals.
- Group 17 is known as halogens and are extremely good oxidising agents. They form ions with a -1 charge known as halides. Metal halides are often crystalline and soluble in water.
- Group 18 consist of inert elements known as noble gases. Due to the complete octet structures, they are generally unreactive and exists as mono-atomic molecules.
- Metals are usually extracted through the reduction of metal ores into the metals using carbon or carbon monoxide. Otherwise they have to be extracted using electrolysis.

Bonding

- There are three major types of bonding: Ionic bonds, covalent bonds and metallic bonds. Dot-and-cross diagrams are often used to show the bonding in ionic and covalent bonds.
- Ionic bonds are formed when electrons are transferred from one atom to another resulting in the formation of positive and negative ions. The electrostatic attractions between the positive and negative ions hold the compound together.
- Ionic bond strength is proportional to the charges of the ions, and inversely proportional the ionic radius of the ions.
- Ionic compounds are usually soluble in water and other polar solvents and conduct electricity easily in molten form. They are usually insoluble in non-polar solvents such as petroleum ether and other organic solvents.
- Covalent bonds are formed by sharing electrons to give an octet structure (usually). There are some circumstances where an octet structure is not formed.

- Covalent compounds usually have lower boiling and melting points due to the weak intermolecular forces of attraction holding molecules together. Their polarity will determine if they are more soluble in polar or non-polar solvents.
- Polarity in covalent compounds is determined by the difference in the electronegativity of the atoms and the orientation of the atoms.
- Metallic bonding occurs in metals, where the nuclei of the metal atoms lie in a sea of delocalised electrons. The electrons can move freely within these molecular orbitals, and so each electron becomes detached from its parent atom. The electrons are said to be delocalised. The metal is held together by the strong forces of attraction between the positive nuclei and the delocalised electrons.

Mole Concept

- Moles are used to measure the amount of a substance in Chemistry. One mole of a compound consist of 6.02×10^{23} molecules of the compound.
- For any compound, 1 mole of the compound will weigh its molecular mass in grams.

Common Chemical Reactions

- Combination chemical reactions: In combination reactions, two or more reactants form one product. The reaction of sodium and chlorine to form sodium chloride.
- Decomposition chemical reactions: Decomposition reactions are really the opposite of combination reactions. In decomposition reactions, a single compound breaks down into two or more simpler substances (elements and/or compounds). The decomposition of water into hydrogen and oxygen gases.
- Single displacement chemical reactions: In single displacement reactions, a more active element displaces another less active element from a compound. For example, if you put a piece of zinc metal into a copper(II) sulfate solution, the zinc displaces the copper. The

reactivity series is as listed, with K being the most reactive and Au being the least:

K>Na>Ca>Mg>Al>Zn>Fe> Pb>H_2>Cu>Hg>Ag>Pt>Au

- Precipitation reactions: The formation of an insoluble solid in a solution is called precipitation.
- Neutralization reactions: The other type of double-displacement reaction is the reaction between an acid and a base. This double-displacement reaction, called a neutralization reaction, forms water.
- Combustion chemical reactions: Combustion reactions occur when a compound, usually one containing carbon, combines with the oxygen gas in the air. This process is commonly called burning. Combustion reactions are also a type of redox reaction.
- Redox chemical reactions: Redox reactions, or reduction-oxidation reactions, are reactions in which electrons are exchanged.
- Condensation reactions: Condensation occurs when two smaller molecules are joined together, with the release of a molecule of water or hydrochloric acid as a by-product.
- Hydrolysis reactions are opposite of condensation reactions, and typically involved the breaking of a larger molecule with the addition of a water molecule into smaller fragments.

Concentrations

- Concentrations in chemistry are often given in mol dm^{-3} or g dm^{-3}.
- 1 mol dm^{-3} = 1 M
- Sometimes, you will see the volumes in L. 1L = 1dm^{-3}.
- For medicine, concentrations are often expressed in mmol dm^{-3}. Just remember that 1000 mmol = 1 mol.

pH Scale

- pH is the measure of the acidity of a solution. It is a logarithmic scale.
- pH = -$\log_{10}$ [H^+]
- The pH scale typically ranges from 1 (acidic) to 14 (alkaline).

- pH only measures the acidity of a solution, and does not indicate the strength of an acid.

Rates of Reaction

- The rate of a reaction is defined as the rate at which products is produced, or the rate which reactants is used up.
- For a zeroth order reaction, the change in the concentration of the reactants will not change the rate of the reaction.
- For a first order reaction, the change in the concentration of the reactant will have a linear proportionate change in the rate of the reaction.
- For a second order reaction, the change in the concentration of the reactant will have an exponential change in the rate of the reaction.
- Rate increases with temperature as the reactant molecules gain more energy, resulting in more effective collisions and increasing the rate of reaction.
- Rate increases with a catalyst as the catalyst lowers the activation energy, resulting in more effective collisions and increasing the rate of reaction.

Chemical Energetics

- Exothermic reactions result in heat energy being released as a product of the reaction. Bond formation is always an exothermic process.
- The enthalpy of an exothermic process is negative.
- Endothermic reactions result in heat energy being absorbed as a reactant of the reaction. Bond breaking in always an endothermic process.
- The enthalpy of an endothermic process is positive.
- A catalyst does not affect the overall enthalpy of a reaction, but will change the activation energy of a reaction.

Hydrocarbons

- Alkanes are saturated hydrocarbons with carbon and hydrogen atoms only. Only single bonds exist in the molecule. They will burn completely in oxygen to form water and carbon dioxide only.
- Alkene and alkynes are unsaturated hydrocarbons with carbon and hydrogen atoms only. At least one double bond exist between carbon atoms in alkenes, and at least one triple bond exist between carbon atoms in alkynes. They will burn completely in oxygen to form water and carbon dioxide only.
- Alkanes have a general formula of C_nH_{2n+2}
- Alkenes have a general formula of C_nH_{2n}
- Alkynes have a general formula of C_nH_{2n-2}
- Short hydrocarbons are often obtained from cracking of long hydrocarbon chains.
- Alkenes and alkynes are often used in addition polymerisation to form useful polymers.
- Isomers have the same molecular formula, but different arrangement of atoms in space.

Biology

Nutrients

- Carbohydrates: Main source of energy in our diets. Mainly digested by amylase.
- Proteins: Source of cellular material for building new cells and growth. Mainly digested by pepsin, trypsin, chymotrypsin in the stomach.
- Fats: Secondary source of energy, also for insulation and protection. Mainly digested by bile salts and lipase.

Digestive System

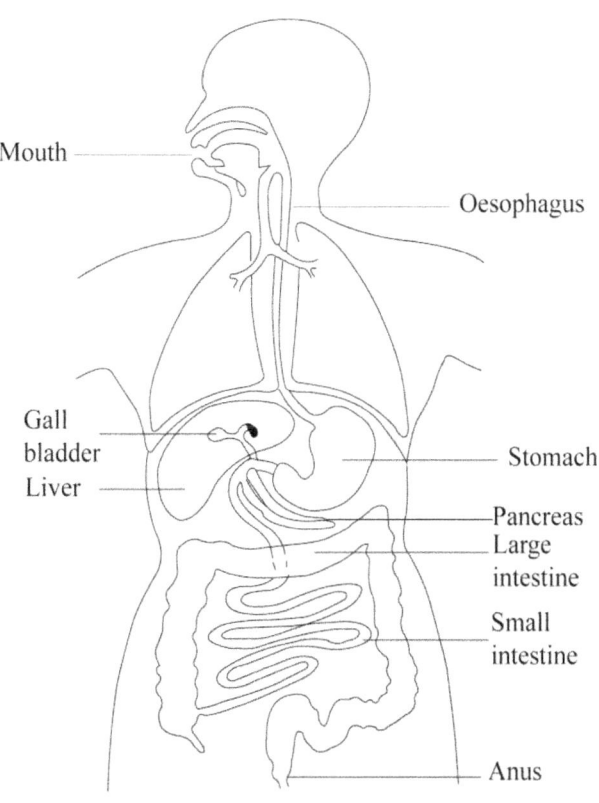

- Digestion in the mouth: Food is chewed to create a larger surface area for the action of enzymes. Saliva is released which contains amylase. Amylase digests starch into smaller sugars (maltose). Further chewing enables swallowing. The food enters the oesophagus.
- Digestion in the stomach: Food enters the stomach from the oesophagus. The walls of our stomach produce gastric juice. This juice contains: A protease enzyme – called pepsin. This digests proteins into amino acids. Hydrochloric acid – this kills bacteria in our food. It creates an acidic environment. Mucus – this protects the wall of our stomach from acid and pepsin. The wall of our stomach is muscular, and churns our food.
- Digestion and absorption in the small intestine: The small intestine has 2 main jobs: (1) To complete the digestion of the food, (2) To absorb the soluble products of digestion into the blood. The food remains in our stomach for a few hours. The proteins are digested. Food leaves our stomach in small squirts into the small intestine.
- Digestion in the small intestine: 3 juices are released:

1. Bile - Produced by the liver.
   o   Stored in the gall bladder.
   o   Released into the small intestine.
   o   2 main things in bile: Alkali to neutralise the stomach acid. Bile salts which convert large fat droplets to small fat droplets – for a large surface area for the enzymes to act on.
   o   There are no enzymes in bile.

2. Pancreatic juice and 3. intestinal juice
   o   Both are released into the small intestine.
   o   Both contain 3 main enzymes:
   o   Amylase to complete the digestion of starch into sugars.
   o   Protease to complete the digestion of proteins into amino acids.
   o   Lipase to break down fats into fatty acids and glycerol.

Respiratory System

Human Respiratory System:

- The human respiratory system is made up of air passages, lungs and the respiratory muscles.
- Nose: most breathing and gas exchange occur through the nose. It is lined by a layer of mucus and hair to trap the dust and germs in the air. It is also supplied with a dense network of blood capillaries to warm the air entering the body.
- Pharynx: Works together with the epiglottis to block the nasal cavity and the trachea during swallowing food, to prevent it from entering the respiratory system.
- Trachea (windpipe): this is a tube that connects the nasal cavity and larynx to the lungs. It is lined with a layer of ciliated epithelium cells and goblet cells which secrete mucus that traps bacteria and dust from inhaled air and gets moved upwards to the larynx by the cilia.
- Bronchi: when the trachea reaches the lungs, it is divided into two tubes, one goes to the right lung and one goes to the left lung. These are called the bronchi. The bronchi are then divided bronchioles that extended deeper into the lungs.
- Alveoli (air sacs): these are tiny bags full of gas; they are present in the lungs in large amounts (several million alveolus in each lung). They give the lungs a much larger surface area for faster diffusion of gases between them and the blood. Each alveolus is supplied with blood capillaries. These come from the pulmonary artery and they contain deoxygenated blood rich in carbon dioxide. The concentration of oxygen is very high inside the alveolus and very low in the blood, so oxygen molecules diffuse from the alveolus to the red blood cells and combine with haemoglobin. At the very same time this occurs, carbon dioxide diffuses from the blood to the alveolus because the concentration of it is very high in the blood and low in the alveolus.
- Diaphragm: this is a sheath of muscles that separates the thoracic cavity from the abdominal cavity. Together with the ribs and the intercostal muscles, it plays a big role in breathing and gas exchange.
- During inhalation, the brain sends electric impulses by nerves to the diaphragm and the intercostal muscles. The diaphragm contracts becoming flatter. The inter-costal muscles also contract and move the ribs in an outer upwards directions. These actions expand the thoracic

cavity making the lungs expand, thus increasing the increasing the volume, with the volume increasing the internal pressure decreases which makes air enter the lungs through the mouth, nose and trachea.

- During exhalation, the diaphragm and the intercostal muscles relax again, contracting the thoracic cavity thus squeezing the air out of the lungs to the trachea and mouth and nose to the atmosphere.

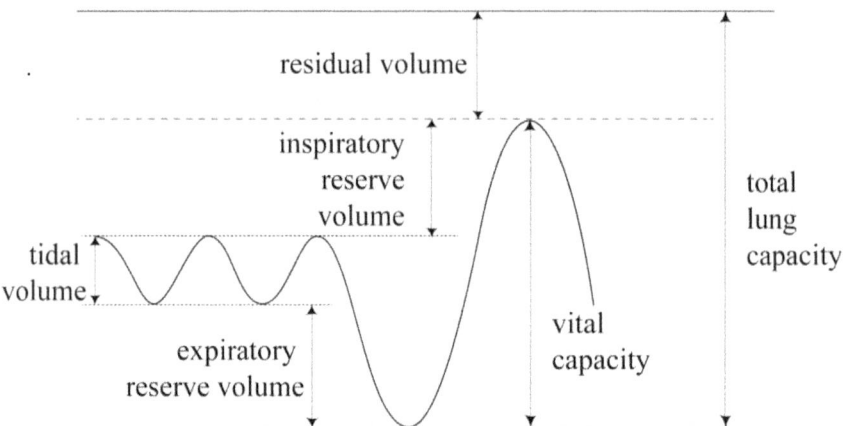

- Aerobic respiration: Glucose is broken down by oxygen to release energy with carbon dioxide and water being produced as by-products of the reaction. Approximately 2900 kJ of energy is released when one mole of glucose is broken down. The released energy is used to make a special energy molecule called Adenosine triphosphate (ATP). ATP is where the energy is stored for use later on by the body.

- Anaerobic respiration is not as efficient as aerobic and only a small amount of energy is released. This is because glucose can only be partially broken down. As well as this inefficiency a poisonous chemical, lactic acid is also produced, if this builds up in the body it stops the muscles from working and causes a cramp. To rid the body of lactic acid oxygen is needed, the amount of oxygen required to break down the lactic acid is referred to as the oxygen debt.

Circulatory System

- Humans have a double circulatory system.
- The heart and blood vessels carry out a transport function. They carry food molecules, water and oxygen to cells and remove waste products such as carbon dioxide in the blood.
- Blood flow in the body: Blood returns from the body to the right atrium. The blood has lost most of the oxygen it carries and is now deoxygenated. The right ventricle pumps the blood along the pulmonary artery to the lungs where it picks up fresh oxygen. It is now oxygenated. The oxygenated blood enters the left side of the heart and is pumped out through the aorta to the body. Once it reaches the capillaries around the body, oxygen diffuses out to the surrounding cells. The deoxygenated blood is carried back towards the heart in the veins. These join up to form the vena cava which is the largest vein.

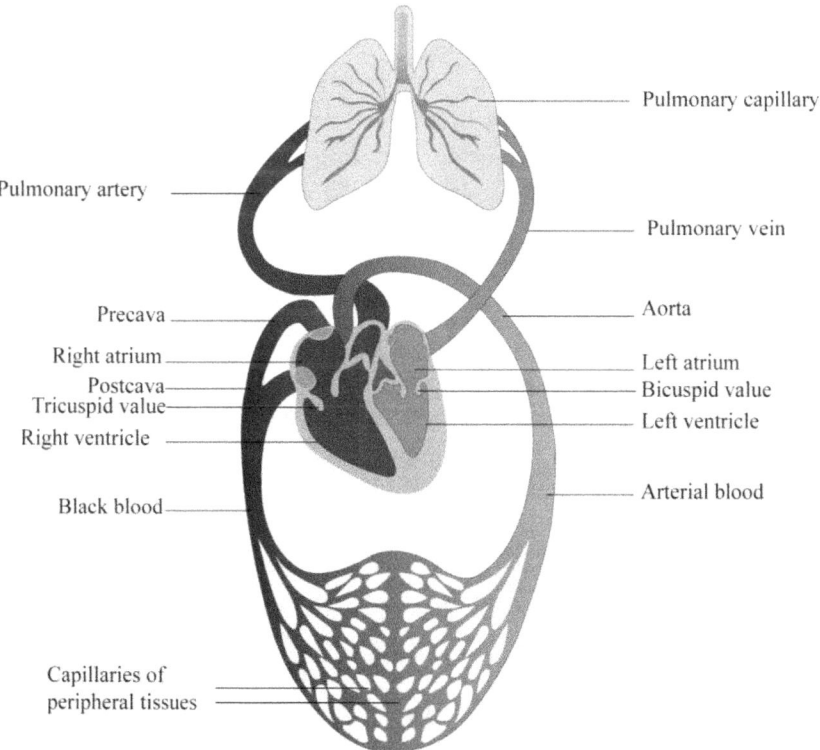

- The four valves in the heart in the order which blood passes through are tricuspid, pulmonary, bicuspid, aortic valve.
- Cardiac output = stroke volume (in mL) x heart rate (beats per minute)
- Blood pressure: written in systolic pressure over diastolic pressure (eg 120/70 mm Hg).
- Blood composition: 55% plasma (water, proteins) , 45% cells (red and white blood cells)

Nervous System

- The nervous system enables humans to react to their surroundings and coordinate their behaviour.
- Information from receptors passes along cells (called neurones) in nerves to the brain.
- Nerve impulses are electrical signals that travel along neurones. Nerve impulses travel at high speed.
- Receptors detect stimuli which include light, sound, changes in position, chemicals, touch, pressure, pain and temperature.
- Sensory neurones – transmit nerve impulses from the receptors to the CNS when a stimulus is detected.
- Motor neurones – transmit nerve impulses from the CNS to effectors, to bring about a response.
- Effectors are muscles or glands.
- The nervous system can be defined into 2 areas: 1. Central nervous system (CNS) consisting of the brain and spinal cord which coordinates the response. 2. Peripheral nervous system (PNS) which consists of nerves connecting the CNS to the rest of the body. Nerves are bundles of motor and sensory neurones.
- Synapses are the connections between neurones. When the impulses reaches the end of the axon it causes a chemical to be released. They are called neurotransmitters. They diffuse across the gap and stimulate the impulse to continue in the next neurone.
- A reflex is a rapid automatic response to a stimulus, which does not involve conscious control. A reflex arc is the route taken by a nerve impulse from receptor to effector via the central nervous system to bring about a reflex action. This involves:

1. A receptor
2. Sensory neurone
3. Relay neurone – a short connecting neurone in the CNS
4. A motor neurone
5. An effector

Excretory System

- Kidneys have an important role in homeostasis. They control the water content of the blood. They control the ion (salt) content of the blood. They remove the urea from the blood.
- Each kidney receives blood from the aorta (via a renal artery). The artery branches into millions of capillaries inside each kidney. Each kidney also contains about one million microscopic tubules, which are responsible for forming urine.

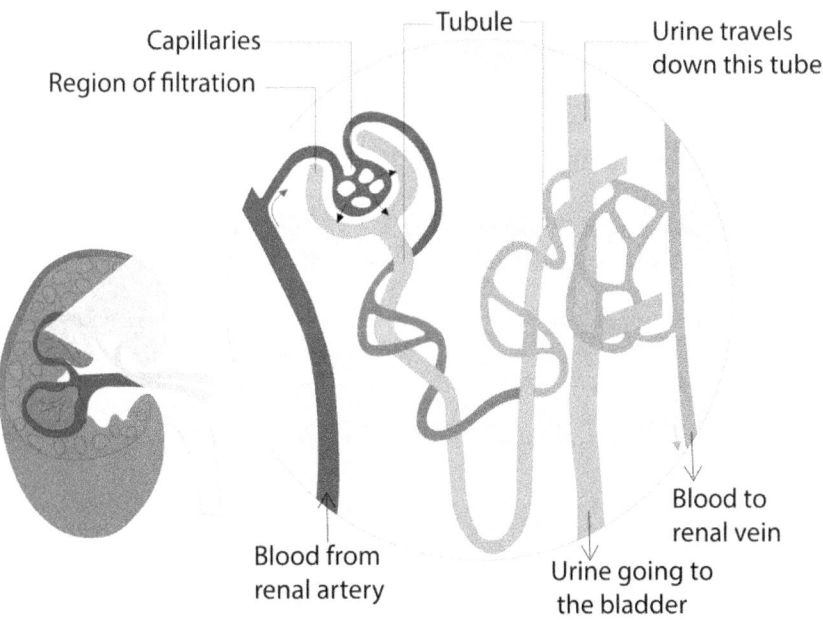

Capillaries

Region of filtration

Tubule

Urine travels down this tube

Blood from renal artery

Urine going to the bladder

Blood to renal vein

- Urine production:
  1. Filtering the blood: Blood enters the capillaries under high pressure. Most of the liquid leaves the blood and enters a tubule. The cells and large molecule remain in the blood. The blood becomes very concentrated.
  2. Reabsorbing all the sugar: All of the sugar is reabsorbed from the tubule, back into the blood by active transport. It moves against a concentration gradient.
  3. Reabsorbing the dissolved ions needed by the body: Some of the ions are also reabsorbed back into the blood by active transport. Some salt is left behind to balance what the body needs.
  4. Reabsorbing as much water as the body needs: Water is reabsorbed into the blood by osmosis. This occurs because there is a much higher solute concentration (lower water concentration) in the blood than in the tubule. The body balances how much water it needs by changing how much water is lost in the urine.
  5. Releasing urine: Urine is released from the kidney. It contains urea, excess ions and water. Urine is stored in the bladder, before being expelled from the body.

Homeostasis

- Homeostasis is the maintenance of a constant internal environment using feedback pathways.

- Some examples of internal environment elements that need to be kept constant include pH of the blood, water potential of blood, CO_2 concentration in blood, body temperature, various salt concentrations.

Endocrine System

- Many processes within the body are coordinated by chemical substances called hormones. Hormones are secreted by glands and are transported to their target organs by the bloodstream. Hormones regulate the functions of many organs and cells.

- Common glands and hormones in the body.

Gland	Hormone	Target organs	Effect
adrenal gland	adrenalin	vital organs, eg liver and heart	Prepares body for action - 'fight or flight'.
ovary	oestrogen	ovaries, uterus, pituitary gland	Controls puberty and the menstrual cycle in females; stimulates production of LH and suppresses the production of FSH in the pituitary gland.
ovary	progesterone	uterus	Maintains the lining of the womb - suppresses FSH production in the pituitary gland.
pancreas	insulin	liver	Controls blood sugar levels.
pituitary gland	anti-diuretic hormone (ADH)	kidney	Controls blood water level by triggering uptake of water in kidneys.
pituitary gland	follicle stimulating hormone (FSH)	ovaries	Triggers egg ripening and oestrogen production in ovaries.
pituitary gland	luteinising hormone (LH)	ovaries	Triggers egg release and progesterone production in ovaries.
testes	testosterone	male reproductive organs	Controls puberty in males.

- Menstrual Cycle
- Hormonal control of menstrual cycle
  - FSH – follicle stimulating hormone
    - Secreted from: pituitary gland
    - Effects: egg matures in ovary
    - Release of oestrogen from ovary
  - Oestrogen
    - Secreted from: ovaries
    - Effects: inhibits release of FSH
    - Causes release of LH
  - LH – luteinising hormone
    - Secreted from: pituitary gland
    - Effects: stimulates release of egg from ovary

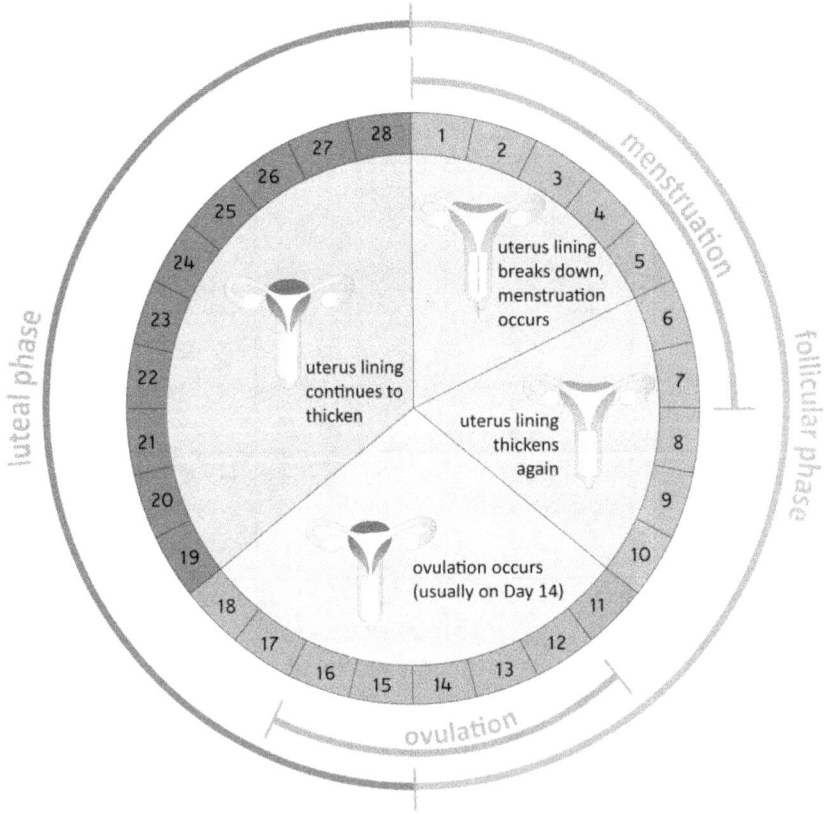

DNA, Genes, Reproduction

- DNA (Deoxyribose nucleic acid) is the chemical found in the nucleus of all cells that
contains the genetic information.
- Chromosomes are thread-like structures made of DNA found in the nucleus
- Genes are small sections of a chromosome that control the characteristics of an organism. Different genes control the development of different characteristics. Genes are passed on from parent to offspring, resulting in offspring having similar characteristics to their parents. Eg eye colour.
- Asexual reproduction: There is no fusion of gametes and only one individual is needed as the parent. There is no mixing of genetic information and so no variation in the offspring. These genetically identical individuals are known as clones.
- Sexual reproduction: Sexual reproduction - the joining (fusion) of male and female gametes. The mixture of the genetic information from two parents leads to variety in the offspring. Genes are passed on in the sex cells (gametes) from which the offspring develop.

Inheritance

- In the nucleus of a typical human body cell there are 23 pairs of chromosomes.
- We inherit one set of 23 from each of our parents. Chromosomes are made from a large molecule called DNA (deoxyribose nucleic acid). DNA has 2 main roles: It can replicate prior to cell division (mitosis or meiosis). Its code is used to synthesise proteins.
- A gene is a small section of DNA. Each gene codes for a particular combination of amino acids which make a specific protein. Some characteristics are controlled by a single gene. Each gene may have different forms called alleles.
- When we are conceived, we receive one copy of each gene from both parents. Therefore we have two copies of every gene, but they may be 2 different alleles. Different combinations of alleles may lead to differences in the characteristic. An allele, which controls the

development of a characteristic when it is present on only one of the chromosomes, is a dominant allele. An allele, which controls the development of characteristics only if the dominant allele is not present, is a recessive allele.

- Punnett Square: Used to calculate the mathematical probability of inheriting a specific trait. This is a simple graphical way of discovering all of the potential combinations of genotypes that can occur in children, given the genotypes of their parents. It also shows us the odds of each of the offspring genotypes occurring.

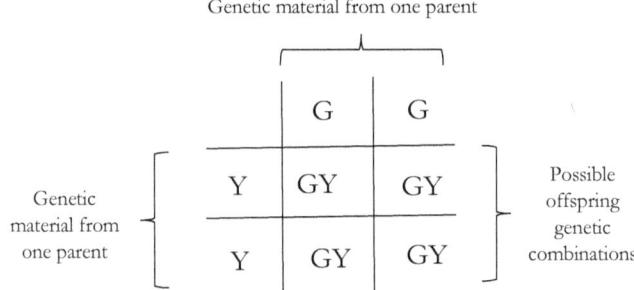

- A pedigree chart is a diagram that shows the occurrence and appearance or phenotypes of a particular gene or organism and its ancestors from one generation to the next. An example is shown below, with males in squares, females in circles, and those affected shaded in black.

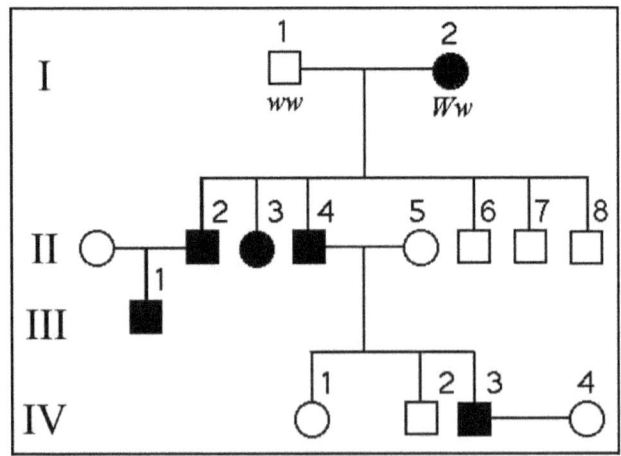

Cell Division

- Mitosis is the type of cell division that leads to growth or repair. When a cell divides by mitosis: two new cells form, each cell is identical to the other one, and the cell they were formed from.
- Stages of Mitosis: parent cell
  1. chromosomes make identical copies of themselves
  2. they line up along the centre
  3. they move apart
  4. two daughter cells form with identical chromosomes to the parent cell
- In meiosis, the cells that are formed have half as many chromosomes as the cell that formed them. Human body cells contain 23 pairs of chromosomes, while human gametes contain 23 single chromosomes.
- The main features of meiosis are: the chromosomes are copied, the cell divides twice, forming four gametes.

Section 3: Writing Task

The writing task is allocated 30 minutes, and must be completed within one side of an A-4 sheet of paper. That is typically about 330 words for a student. Most students will be able to complete writing their essays in 15 minutes, allowing another 15 minutes for question selection, essay planning and checking.

Essay Checklist

Each essay is marked by two markers and the average is taken for the final score. If the two scores deviate too far, a third marker is brought in to moderate the score.

The BMAT essay markers are looking for the following in your essays which you should strive to include:

- Has the candidate answered the question?
- Are the terms properly and correctly defined, if required?
- Has the candidate explained the proposition and explained the implications?
- Were there reasonable counter-arguments?
- Were there suggestions of how conflicts between arguments could be resolved?
- Are the thoughts organised clearly?
- Are the arguments logical?
- Is there good use of general knowledge in the essays?
- Have candidates expressed themselves clearing using concise, correct and compelling English.

Essay Selection

You will be given a choice of four questions to choose from. Each question is usually a statement, a quote or a paragraph on a philosophical question which you would have to argue for, or against, depending on the question.

Read each question carefully and mark out key details of each question. Every question will have specific instructions for you to define or explain the propositions, and argue your essay in a particular manner. Each essay will always have three components and will require you to argue from multiple points of view. Highlight these clearly to make sure you answer the question.

At least one of the questions will be related to the biomedical field, for example related to medical ethics, animal treatment and use of drugs. It would be useful if you have spent some time reading up articles and various argument on the following themes:

- Animal cruelty
- Nature conservation
- Euthanasia
- Patient consent
- Doctor-assisted suicide
- Affordable healthcare in society
- Use of experimental drugs
- Role of medicine in society

Usually there will be a question on science and technology, but not always. Many of these questions are also intentionally tied into biomedical questions, such as use of technology in biomedical science. Science and technology questions are often more general and discuss effect of science and technology on humanity. It would be useful if you have spent some time reading up articles and various argument on the following themes:

- Scientific knowledge
- Advances in biomedical technology
- Science and society
- Science, technology and human development

You should choose a question which you are comfortable with and able to do all the following:

1. Define the terms required in the question confidently;
2. Generate least three ideas in favour of the argument;
3. Generate least three ideas against the argument;
4. Provide one example for each idea where applicable.

Essay Structure and Style

It is challenging to prove to the examiners how good you are while keeping to the page limit of one side of the A-4 sized sheet. You would need to be concise, efficient and clear in your language. Do not ramble, go about in circles or use unnecessary words.

We suggest a four-paragraph structure which is simple and easy to fit within the page limit:

1. Introduction and definitions – short, simple, two or three sentences.
2. Arguments for – At least two arguments, good to have one example. Your arguments should be from different points of view where possible (example: legal aspects, practical aspects, cultural aspects). You should also include one implication of the proposition. Typically 4 sentences in this paragraph.
3. Arguments against – Same as arguments for.
4. Conclusion – Analyse both arguments and come to a conclusion with your stand. Resolve conflicts between arguments and propose solutions. About two or three sentences in this paragraph.

So in terms of the number of sentences for each paragraph, it is about 2-4-4-3.

Your sentences should be varied but concise. Long sentences are useful to link arguments together but can be difficult to read. Students also tend to put too many ideas in a long sentence. Shorter sentences are clearer and concise, but result in choppy essays if overused.

Avoid jargons, technical abbreviations and big words unless you absolutely need to. While marks are given for good language, the ability to communicate your ideas clearly are more important.

Be confident in your arguments and do not use ambiguous words and sentences. Sentences such as "I believe that the assertion is flawed because…" show more confidence in your arguments as compared to "The assertion might be wrong…"

It is important that your essay is writing in correct English. Be mindful of your grammar and sentence structures to provide for an easy-to-read essay. Varied sentence structures, good use of vocabulary, proper use of grammar and correct spelling will help you get a good essay score.

Worked Example

Mentol wellbeing has nothing to do with physical wellbeing. What do you take this statement to mean? Develop a counter-argument that refuses the author's view. Do you believe that a healthy mind equals a healthy body?

The statement implies that there is no relationship between the physical health and the mental health of a person.

Argument for	Argument against
Can be physically healthy and mentally ill at the same time. [Argument using examples]	Mental wellbeing will affect how a person treats his body and hence affect physical well-being. [Argument using examples]
Psychiatric medicine is a distinct branch of medicine. [Argument by quoting experts]	Research showing relationship between mental and physical health. [Experts]
Physical impairment does not lead to mental problems. [Reversing the argument]	

Essay Arguments

Animal testing should be banned.

Argument for	Argument against
Animals have rights not to be harmed.	Animal research necessary to save human lives.
Research can be done without animal testing.	Animal rights are of less moral worth than human rights.
Send a positive social message.	Animal research is only used when other research methods are not suitable.

Animals should have the same rights as humans.

Argument for	Argument against
Animals are intrinsically worthy of rights because they are sentient.	Animals are not moral agents
Animals are equal to human beings.	Animals have no interests or rationality
Even if we did think that animals were less intelligent than humans beings they should be protected by rights	Most rights have no bearing for animals

Euthanasia should be allowed.

Argument for	Argument against
Allowing people to 'die with dignity' is kinder than forcing them to continue their lives with suffering.	Alternative treatments are available, such as palliative care and hospices.
Every patient has a right to choose when to die.	Opening the doors to voluntary euthanasia could lead to non-voluntary and involuntary euthanasia.
Euthanasia can be safely regulated by government legislation.	Cannot be completely controlled.

Human cloning should be banned.

Argument for	Argument against
Cloning is unsafe.	Allows for the elimination of some diseases.
Cloning is playing God.	Clones have awareness and are still individuals.
Cloning treats children as objects.	Cloning should be allowed for people who cannot have children.

Science as a threat to society.

Argument for	Argument against
Manipulation of life is playing god.	Lives can be more fulfilling.
Science enable more destruction.	Science is only a tool.
Science has created new methods to control the lives of the citizenry.	Science saves and improves lives.

Banning the development of genetically modified organisms.

Argument for	Argument against
Genetically modified food is too new and little researched to be allowed for public use.	Genetically modified food is no different from any other scientific advance, thus should be legal to use.
Genetically modified food is a danger to eco-systems.	Genetically modified organisms can solve the problem of food supply in the developing world.
GMOs would create too much dependency on biotechnology companies	Genetically modified organisms will prevent starvation due to global climate changes.

Legalising sale of human organs.

Argument for	Argument against
Recognize the benefits of individuals who are able to pay for their healthcare doing so.	Allowing the sale of organs will harm state-financed health services and create a two-tier system.
Legalising the sale of organs will eradicate the black market and ensure safer transplants.	Allowing the sale of human organs in the First World will impact negatively on the Third World.
People should have rights over their own body and body parts.	Individuals do not have an inviolable right of property over their organs.

Parents should be able to choose the sex of their children.

Argument for	Argument against
Gender selection will prevent incidents of infanticide	Pre-selection of gender uses expensive medical care for frivolous purposes
Parents should have freedom of choice	Children should not be designed to specifications
Sex-specific, generic diseases can be avoided	Science should not play God.

Wild animals should not be kept in captivity.

Argument for	Argument against
Wild animals in zoos suffer unnecessarily	Zoos act as educational tools
Zoos encourage the use of animals as mere entertainment	Zoos help to protect endangered species
Wild animals belong in their natural habitat	Zoos permit longer, more fruitful scientific research

Suggested readings

Here are some topics which you might want to spend some time to read up to better prepare yourself for possible examination questions.

- Abortion
- Alternative Medicine
- Animal rights
- Artificial insemination
- Artificial life
- Assisted suicide
- Body modification
- Chimeras
- Cloning
- Confidentiality (medical records)
- Consent
- Contraception (birth control)
- Cryonics
- Disability
- Eugenics
- Euthanasia (human, non-human animal)
- Exorcism
- Faith Healing
- Genetically modified food
- Genetically modified organism
- Genomics
- Human cloning
- Human enhancement
- Human genetic engineering
- Life extension
- Life support
- Medical malpractice
- Overtreatment
- Organ donation
- Organ transplant
- Pain management
- Patients' Bill of Rights
- Placebo
- Quality of Life (Healthcare)
- Recreational drug use
- Reproductive rights
- Reproductive technology
- Stem cell research
- Vaccination controversy

Visit **http://www.bmat.sg** to get more resources and download free essays.

www.ingramcontent.com/pod-product-compliance
Lightning Source LLC
Chambersburg PA
CBHW070843180526
45168CB00002B/949